HERBS FOR DERMATITIS BITES

Nature's Soothing Solutions: Unlocking The Power To Conquer Insect   Disease Naturally

DR. JEREMY ALLEY

Disclaimer:

The information provided in this book, is intended for general informational purposes only and should not be considered as professional advice.

The author has made every effort to ensure the accuracy of the information presented. However, readers are advised to consult with a qualified healthcare professional before attempting any herbal remedies or making significant changes to their wellness routine. Individual health conditions vary, and what may be suitable for one person may not be appropriate for another.

It is important to note that the author is not in any endorsement deal, partnership, or affiliation with any organization, brand, or company mentioned in this book. Any references to specific products or services are based on the author's personal experience or general knowledge and do not imply an endorsement or promotion of those products or services.

Contents

Overview

We explore the realm of herbal treatments for dermatitis bites in this in-depth guide, providing insightful information and helpful tips to lessen the pain brought on by these unpleasant skin disorders.

Greetings of Welcome

We extend a hearty welcome to readers looking for safe, all-natural remedies for bites caused by dermatitis. Our goal as we set out on this journey together is to offer you useful advice and doable solutions to help you stop the itching, redness, and inflammation brought on by dermatitis bites.

The Book's Objective

This book's mission is to arm readers with information about herbal treatments for dermatitis bites. Readers can take proactive measures to manage and mitigate the symptoms connected with these bothersome skin irritations by learning the underlying reasons and implementing herbal treatments.

Knowing What Causes Dermatitis Bites

Understanding the nature and triggers of dermatitis bites is essential to combating them effectively. The term "dermatitis" describes an inflammation of the skin that is frequently accompanied by swelling, redness, and itching. Dermatitis can result from bites from a variety of sources, such as allergies and insects, therefore determining the precise form of dermatitis is crucial for tailored therapy.

The Value of Herbal Remedies

Herbal remedies provide a comprehensive and all-natural method of treating dermatitis bites. Herbal medicines are frequently milder on the skin while still offering effective relief, in contrast to some conventional treatments that may have adverse consequences. Comprehending the significance of integrating herbal remedies into your skincare regimen is imperative for fostering recuperation and averting recurrent episodes of dermatitis bites.

We will examine particular herbal medicines, useful advice, and lifestyle changes that can support an all-encompassing and long-lasting approach to treating dermatitis bites as we progress through the upcoming chapters. The knowledge on these pages is meant to help you on your journey to better and more radiant skin, regardless of whether you are addressing a recent bite or seeking long-term prevention.

CHAPTER ONE

COMMUNICATION WITH DERMATITIS BITES

Bites that result in dermatitis include a variety of skin reactions brought on by bug bites. Those who are bitten by them frequently experience discomfort because of redness, swelling, and itching. Finding appropriate herbal remedies to treat dermatitis bites requires first understanding their nature.

What Are Bites From Dermatitis?

Inflammatory reactions that happen when specific insects bite the skin are referred to as dermatitis bites.

These bites have the potential to cause allergic reactions, which can manifest as swelling, redness, and itching. To find the right herbal treatments for relief, it's critical to distinguish dermatitis bites from other skin diseases.

Typical Reasons And Signs

To effectively treat dermatitis bites, it is essential to investigate their typical causes and symptoms. Oftentimes, insects such as bedbugs, fleas, ticks, and mosquitoes are to blame.

Although the symptoms can vary, itching, redness, and the development of tiny bumps or blisters are frequently present. Identifying the precise cause and symptoms facilitates the customization of herbal remedies for the best outcomes.

Types Of Bites From Dermatitis

There are several types of dermatitis bites, and each one has its own set of difficulties for the person afflicted. This portion of the book explores the various kinds of bug bites and what makes them unique. People can treat the various symptoms of dermatitis bites by using specialized herbal remedies if they are aware of the unique characteristics of each type.

Recognizing Various Insect Bite Types

Finding the best herbal remedies for bug bites requires accurate identification. This chapter offers information on how to differentiate between various insect bite types based on symptoms and appearance. Equipped with this understanding, people can choose herbal medicines with confidence that are unique to the type of insect bite they have experienced.

To sum up, this book is an invaluable tool for anyone looking for natural remedies to ease the pain from dermatitis bites. By delving further into the nature of these bites and offering guidance on potent herbal remedies, readers may take a natural and all-encompassing approach to managing and resolving the issues related to dermatitis bites.

CHAPTER TWO

USE OF HERBS TO TREAT DERMATITIS BITES

Bite dermatitis can cause irritation and discomfort, and treating the condition effectively is generally necessary to reduce symptoms. In addition to providing relief from itching, irritation, and redness without the possible side effects associated with some conventional treatments, herbal therapies offer a natural and comprehensive approach to managing dermatitis bites.

The Potential Of Herbal Treatments

Because of their therapeutic qualities, herbs have been used in traditional medicine for millennia. Their bioactive ingredients and natural chemicals have shown antibacterial, anti-inflammatory, and antipruritic properties that make them particularly useful in the treatment of dermatitis bites. By using the power of herbal treatments, people can treat skin diseases in a sustainable and friendly way.

Advantages Of Using Herbal Remedies

Choosing herbal remedies for dermatitis bites has several advantages. Herbal medicines are generally less harmful than synthetic pharmaceuticals, which makes them appropriate for those with sensitive skin. In addition, a lot of herbs provide nutritional components that support healthy skin in addition to their medicinal qualities. Herbal remedies are holistic in that they treat the underlying causes as well as the symptoms, promoting a whole healing process.

Safety Points To Remember

Although most people think that herbal medicines are harmless, it's important to be cautious and aware of any potential allergies or sensitivities. Certain plants can cause negative reactions in some people, which is why patch tests should always be performed before using a herb widely. It is advisable to speak with a healthcare provider or herbalist, particularly for people who already have medical concerns or are taking additional

The use of herbs to treat dermatitis bites provides a safe, all-natural way to control symptoms. To fully utilize herbal remedies for dermatitis bites, it is essential to comprehend their effectiveness, recognize all of their advantages, and make sure that safety precautions are taken.

CHAPTER THREE

ESSENTIAL HERBS FOR BITES OF DERMATITIS

Bite dermatitis can be painful, resulting in redness, swelling, and itching. Herbal medicines provide a natural, all-encompassing method of symptom relief and healing, in contrast to the many conventional treatments accessible. This thorough guide covers a variety of important herbs that are well-known for helping with dermatitis bites.

Calendula: A Natural Calming Plant

The marigold flower is the source of calendula, which is well known for its calming qualities. It's a useful plant for dermatitis bites because of its anti-inflammatory and antibacterial properties. Calendula-infused lotions and ointments can be applied to alleviate the irritation caused by bug bites and dermatitis by reducing redness and inflammation.

Chamomile: A Calm Restorer

Another herbal cure that is moderate and soothing for dermatitis bites is chamomile. Itching and pain can be lessened by chamomile's soothing and anti-inflammatory qualities. For calming relief, apply chamomile-infused oils topically to troubled regions or use compresses made of chamomile tea.

Lavender: Fragrant Soothing

In addition to its pleasant scent, lavender has medicinal qualities that make it helpful for bites caused by dermatitis. Because of its antibacterial and anti-inflammatory properties, lavender oil helps mend damaged skin and lessens irritation. For aromatic alleviation, apply a few drops of diluted lavender oil to the affected region.

Aloe Vera: Refreshing and Inducing Pain

Aloe vera is a multipurpose plant that has anti-inflammatory and cooling qualities. The leaves gel can be used topically to treat dermatitis bites to calm the skin, lessen inflammation, and hasten recovery. The instant respite from insect bite pain is offered by aloe vera's inherent cooling effect.

The Natural Antiseptic Of Tea Tree Oil

Tea tree oil works well as a herbal cure for dermatitis bites because it has strong antibacterial and antimicrobial qualities. Applying diluted tea tree oil to the afflicted region can help soothe the skin, lessen inflammation, and stop infection. To prevent skin irritation, it is imperative to use tea tree oil sparingly and to dilute it properly.

Strong Anti-Bacterial Herb: Neem

The neem tree yields neem, a strong antibacterial plant. It is useful for treating dermatitis bites because of its antibacterial and anti-inflammatory qualities. Neem oil or lotions infused with neem can be applied topically to relieve irritation and itching while also promoting healing and preventing infection.

Additional Helpful Herbs

In addition to the herbs listed above, several additional herbs can provide treatment for dermatitis bites. Plantain can be administered topically to lessen itching because of its anti-inflammatory qualities.

 Applying witch hazel, which has astringent qualities, to the afflicted area can also help. Furthermore, a strong herbal remedy for dermatitis bites can be made by combining calendula, chamomile, and lavender.

Herbal remedies for dermatitis bites provide a safe, all-natural way to reduce symptoms and encourage recovery. With their distinct qualities, these herbs can be used singly or in combination to effectively relieve irritation, redness, and inflammation.

CHAPTER FOUR

SUMMARY FOR SKIN HEALTH

Achieving and maintaining good skin is a complex process, and diet is essential to its maintenance. A healthy diet is crucial for maintaining general health, and the need for adequate nutrition increases when it comes to treating dermatitis and bug bites.

The Value Of A Well-Balanced Diet

Maintaining the body's many processes, particularly those linked to skin health, requires a balanced diet. The body gets vital vitamins, minerals, and antioxidants from a balanced diet, all of which support the preservation of good skin. The body's capacity to heal itself and protect itself from outside stimulants is weakened by a diet deficient in essential nutrients, which may exacerbate the symptoms of dermatitis.

Vitamins That Promote Skin Health

Several nutrients are essential for maintaining good skin and treating bug bite dermatitis. For instance, vitamin E is well-known for its antioxidant qualities and capacity to save the skin from oxidative damage. Flaxseeds and fish oil are good sources of omega-3 fatty acids, which hydrate skin and reduce inflammation. Another important nutrient that helps the skin repair and strengthens the immune system is zinc.

Foods To Take And Leave Out

Including specific foods in your diet can help treat insect-bites-induced dermatitis. Antioxidant-rich foods, like fruits and vegetables, can aid in the reduction of inflammation and neutralization of free radicals. Foods high in omega-3, such as walnuts, chia seeds, and fatty fish, help moisturize the skin and lessen irritation.

Including foods high in zinc, such as quinoa, lentils, and pumpkin seeds, can also help with the healing process.

On the other hand, items that might worsen dermatitis symptoms should be avoided. particular people may be more susceptible to particular allergens, such as gluten or dairy, which might irritate their skin.

To manage dermatitis and avoid recurrent bug bite reactions, it can be quite important to keep an eye on your diet and identify potential trigger foods.

An essential part of treating dermatitis brought on by insect bites is preserving healthy skin via diet.

The skin's capacity to repair and protect itself from future irritation can be enhanced by eating a balanced diet that consists of a range of foods high in nutrients.

People who are aware of the connection between nutrition and skin health are better able to manage and prevent dermatitis by making educated dietary decisions.

CHAPTER FIVE

HERBAL APPLICATIONS AND RECIPES

There are several uses for herbal remedies for dermatitis bites, all of which capitalize on the medicinal qualities of particular plants. These treatments are frequently made as salves, balms, compresses, bath mixtures, and sprays, giving users a variety of external application options.

Botanical Balms And Salves

Making herbal salves and balms is a common way to treat bites from dermatitis. It is common practice to infuse ingredients like calendula, chamomile, and lavender into carrier oils like coconut or olive oil. Beeswax is then mixed with this infusion to create a calming balm that may be administered topically to afflicted areas. These herbs were picked because of their ability to reduce inflammation and promote skin healing.

Herbal Compresses That Are Calm

Compresses made of herbs provide inflamed skin with instant relief. To make an herbal infusion, steep a mixture of herbs, such as chamomile, witch hazel, and comfrey, in hot water. A cloth is soaked in the infusion and used as a compress for the affected areas once it has cooled to a tolerable temperature. This lessens swelling and eases the itchiness brought on by dermatitis bites.

Blends Of Herbs For Baths

A holistic approach to treating dermatitis symptoms is offered by herbal baths. Herbs that relieve itching and aid in skin healing, such as oatmeal, calendula, and Epsom salts, can be added to a warm bath. Herbal baths are a great complement to the dermatitis care regimen since the blend of these herbs has a relaxing and anti-inflammatory impact on the skin.

Homemade Herbal Itch Relief Spray

A homemade herbal spray with ingredients like peppermint, lavender essential oil, and aloe vera can be made for on-the-go treatment. These ingredients are combined with water and kept in a spray bottle for easy application whenever it gets itchy. Aloe vera has a cooling effect, and the spray's anti-itch and anti-inflammatory qualities are enhanced with peppermint and lavender.

Herbal Concoctions For Internal Assistance

In addition, internal support is essential for dermatitis management. You can drink tea made from nettles, calendula, and dandelion infusions. The selection of these herbs is based on their capacity to enhance the body's general inflammatory response and foster internal skin health.

Frequent use of herbal infusions supports a holistic strategy for controlling dermatitis bites by balancing exterior applications.

Herbal remedies provide a holistic and natural substitute for pharmaceutical treatments for dermatitis bites. Herbal remedies are incredibly adaptable; from salves and compresses to bath mixtures and internal infusions, people can customize their regimen according to their tastes and the intensity of their symptoms. By incorporating these herbal remedies into a skincare regimen, you can help promote skin healing and ease discomfort.

CHAPTER SIX

ADVICE ON LIFESTYLE FOR BITES OF DERMATITIS

Bites that cause dermatitis can be excruciating and distressing, and they are frequently caused by insect bites or contact with specific allergens. Adopting a comprehensive strategy that includes lifestyle modifications is necessary for managing and reducing the symptoms of dermatitis bites. You may reduce the negative effects of dermatitis bites on your skin and general health by implementing practical methods into your everyday routine.

Steer Clear Of Triggers

Finding and avoiding triggers that could make dermatitis bites worse is an essential part of controlling the illness. Exposure to specific plants, insects, or environmental conditions are common triggers. You may lessen the chance of coming into touch with these triggers and, as a result, the frequency of dermatitis bites by being aware of your surroundings and actions.

Keeping Up Adequate Hygiene

Dermatitis bites can be prevented and managed with strict hygienic practices. To eliminate irritants and lessen inflammation, wash and cleanse the afflicted regions regularly. Maintaining skin health can be aided by avoiding harsh chemicals and using moderate, fragrance-free soaps. Additionally, avoiding secondary infections from scratching can be achieved by keeping your nails neat and short.

Clothes Selections For Prevention

Wearing the appropriate clothes might help a lot in avoiding dermatitis bites. When going anywhere where there's a chance of getting bitten by a bug, wear long sleeves, slacks, and closed shoes. Additionally helpful may be wearing light-colored clothing, which might deter certain insects from finding you appealing. Think about using essential oils or herbal repellents with proven insect-repelling qualities to your clothing.

Establishing A Pest-Free Ambience

The first step in avoiding dermatitis bites is to create a pest-free atmosphere. To keep insects out of your living areas, choose natural treatments like plant-based repellents or herbal therapies. Maintain your outside spaces properly by getting rid of any standing water and any places where insects might breed. Using natural pest control techniques can assist in reducing the environment that attracts pests that cause dermatitis.

Managing and avoiding dermatitis bites can be greatly aided by implementing these lifestyle changes. People can relieve the discomfort of dermatitis bites and improve the health of their skin by taking proactive measures to prevent triggers, maintaining good hygiene, choosing clothing wisely, and keeping their environment pest-free.

CHAPTER SEVEN

CASE RESEARCH

Examining case studies offers important information on how well herbal remedies work for dermatitis bites. These studies explore real-world situations and describe the experiences of people who have turned to herbal treatments for healing. We can better comprehend the variety of dermatitis bites and the particular difficulties that each encounters by looking at particular situations.

Experiences In Real Life With Herbal Remedies

This section explores first-hand stories from people who used herbal treatments to treat their dermatitis bites. These first-hand accounts provide insight into the use, efficacy, and general effects of herbal remedies. Our goal in sharing these narratives is to present a complete picture of the various ways that people incorporate herbal treatments into their daily routines for managing dermatitis.

Achievement Stories

Success tales demonstrate the beneficial effects of using herbal remedies for dermatitis bites. These personal accounts highlight situations in which people have used herbal medicines in conjunction with their skincare routines to find relief, improvement, or resolution of their dermatitis symptoms.

Success stories motivate those looking for more natural and alternative dermatitis management techniques.

Difficulties And How They Were Solved

A fair viewpoint necessitates addressing the drawbacks of applying herbal remedies for dermatitis bites. This section examines the challenges people may run into when using herbal treatments, including differences in efficacy, individual preferences, or experiences with trial and error.

By drawing attention to these difficulties, we can gain a deeper understanding of the intricacies involved in managing herbal dermatitis and discover how people get past roadblocks to find relief.

CHAPTER EIGHT

INCLUDING NATURAL SOLUTIONS IN EVERYDAY LIFE

Dermatitis bites can be a chronic and painful condition for which there are frequently good herbal remedies. By incorporating these solutions into your routine, you can greatly reduce and avoid the discomfort associated with dermatitis. Calendula, chamomile, and lavender are among the herbs with anti-inflammatory and calming qualities that can be used in a variety of ways to relieve dermatitis bite symptoms.

Including Herbs In Your Daily Routine

A useful strategy for preventing dermatitis bites is to include herbal treatments in your regular skincare regimen. The itching and redness associated with dermatitis can be relieved by using herbal-infused creams, lotions, or oils that contain substances like witch hazel, tea tree oil, or aloe vera. Applying these herbal remedies regularly will help preserve skin health and lessen the frequency of dermatitis flare-ups.

Making First Aid Kits With Herbs

Putting together an herbal first aid pack will help prevent dermatitis bites by being proactive. It can be helpful to include medicinal plants such as calendula, neem, and turmeric in cream, ointment, or tincture form. You can use these herbal treatments directly to problematic areas to aid in healing and reduce inflammation.

When assistance is needed, having a fully supplied herbal first aid kit guarantees that supplies will be on hand.

Disseminating Herbal Knowledge To Others

Spreading knowledge about the advantages of using herbal remedies for dermatitis bites can promote a feeling of well-being throughout the community. By imparting information about certain herbs, their uses, and the value of herbal treatments in the treatment of dermatitis, people can become more proactive with their skin care. Promoting the sharing of herbal knowledge among neighbors can help to establish a supporting network for those with dermatitis problems.

Herbal remedies can help avoid and effectively manage dermatitis bites.

You can prevent and manage dermatitis bites by combining them into your skincare routine, making herbal first aid kits, and teaching people about them. People can find healing and promote a holistic approach to skin health by embracing the power of nature.

CHAPTER NINE

STRATEGIES FOR PREVENTION

A key component of treating dermatitis is preventing bites from the illness. This section looks at a few different ways to prevent typical triggers that result in insect bites. Practical steps to reduce the risk of bites include wearing long sleeves and pants in pest-prone locations, applying insect repellents, and staying indoors during insect peak hours.

Steer Clear Of Common Triggers

Effective avoidance of dermatitis bites requires knowledge of the triggers. Common offenders include fleas, ticks, mosquitoes, and other insects. People can drastically lower their exposure to these insects and their chance of getting dermatitis by recognizing the particular environmental factors that draw them in and implementing preventative measures.

Using Herbs In Everyday Living To Prevent

Adding these herbs into your daily routine can help maintain healthy skin and increase your resistance to insect bites in addition to exterior protective measures. Taking anti-inflammatory herbal teas, like those containing peppermint or chamomile, can offer an additional line of defense from within. Furthermore, applying body washes and shampoos containing herbal infusions might help the skin form a barrier of defense.

Herbal remedies for dermatitis bites provide a comprehensive strategy for controlling and averting the pain brought on by bug bites. People can improve their overall skin health and lessen the effects of insect-bites-induced dermatitis by learning the triggers, using topical herbal therapies, and implementing preventive measures.

Safety Instructions

When handling bites from dermatitis, safety must come first. It's crucial to perform a patch test to rule out any adverse responses before trying any herbal therapies. This entails dabbing a tiny patch of skin with the herbal solution and keeping an eye out for any unfavorable reactions. A healthcare provider should also be consulted, particularly if the person is pregnant or has pre-existing medical issues.

Take Care When Applying Herbal Treatments

Herbal treatments can help with dermatitis bites, but there are some things to watch out for to make sure you use them safely and effectively. Pregnant individuals or those with underlying health issues should consult with a healthcare professional before incorporating herbal solutions into their treatment plan. To prevent any negative effects, it is essential to be aware of possible interactions between herbal remedies and medications.

Moreover, it is essential to follow the recommended dosage and application instructions for each herbal remedy. Excessive use or misuse of herbal solutions may lead to undesirable effects. Individuals should also be cautious about sourcing herbal products from reputable sources to ensure their purity and quality.

Consulting With A Healthcare Professional

Before embarking on any herbal remedy for dermatitis bites, consulting with a healthcare professional is strongly advised. Healthcare professionals can provide personalized guidance based on an individual's health history, allergies, and current medications. They can also offer insights into potential interactions between herbal remedies and conventional treatments.

During the consultation, individuals can discuss their symptoms, the severity of the dermatitis bites, and any previous experiences with herbal remedies. This collaborative approach ensures a well-rounded understanding of the individual's health and enables the healthcare professional to recommend suitable herbal solutions.

while herbal remedies can offer valuable relief for dermatitis bites, it is imperative to prioritize safety by following established guidelines and consulting with healthcare professionals.

These precautions ensure that individuals can effectively manage dermatitis bites with the confidence that their chosen herbal solutions are both safe and beneficial for their specific circumstances.

CONCLUSION

In conclusion, herbal solutions offer a viable and natural alternative for managing dermatitis bites. Calendula, chamomile, aloe vera, tea tree oil, and comfrey are among the herbal remedies that can provide relief from itching, and inflammation, and promote the healing of affected skin. Integrating these remedies into skincare routines can contribute to a holistic and gentle approach to dermatitis management.

Recap Of Important Ideas

Dermatitis bites result from contact with allergens or irritants, causing inflammation and discomfort.

Herbal remedies such as calendula, chamomile, aloe vera, tea tree oil, and comfrey offer natural solutions for dermatitis management.

Each herbal remedy has unique properties, such as anti-inflammatory, antimicrobial, or cell-regenerating, contributing to their effectiveness in soothing and healing the skin.

explore herbal solutions for dermatitis bites, it's essential to approach these remedies with an open mind and a commitment to consistent application. Nature's healing power often requires patience, so persistence in utilizing herbal treatments can lead to long-term relief and improved skin health.

Final Thoughts

In the realm of dermatitis management, herbal solutions provide a gentle and holistic approach that aligns with the body's natural healing processes. By harnessing the therapeutic properties of plants like calendula, chamomile, aloe vera, tea tree oil, and comfrey, individuals can find comfort and relief from the itching and inflammation associated with dermatitis bites.

Embracing these herbal remedies reflects a commitment to a more natural and harmonious relationship with our skin's well-being.